Keto Diet Cookbook for Moments of Relax

50 Tasty and Delicious Recipes for your Snack, but staying Healthy. Ideal for Women Over 50

Rose Pope

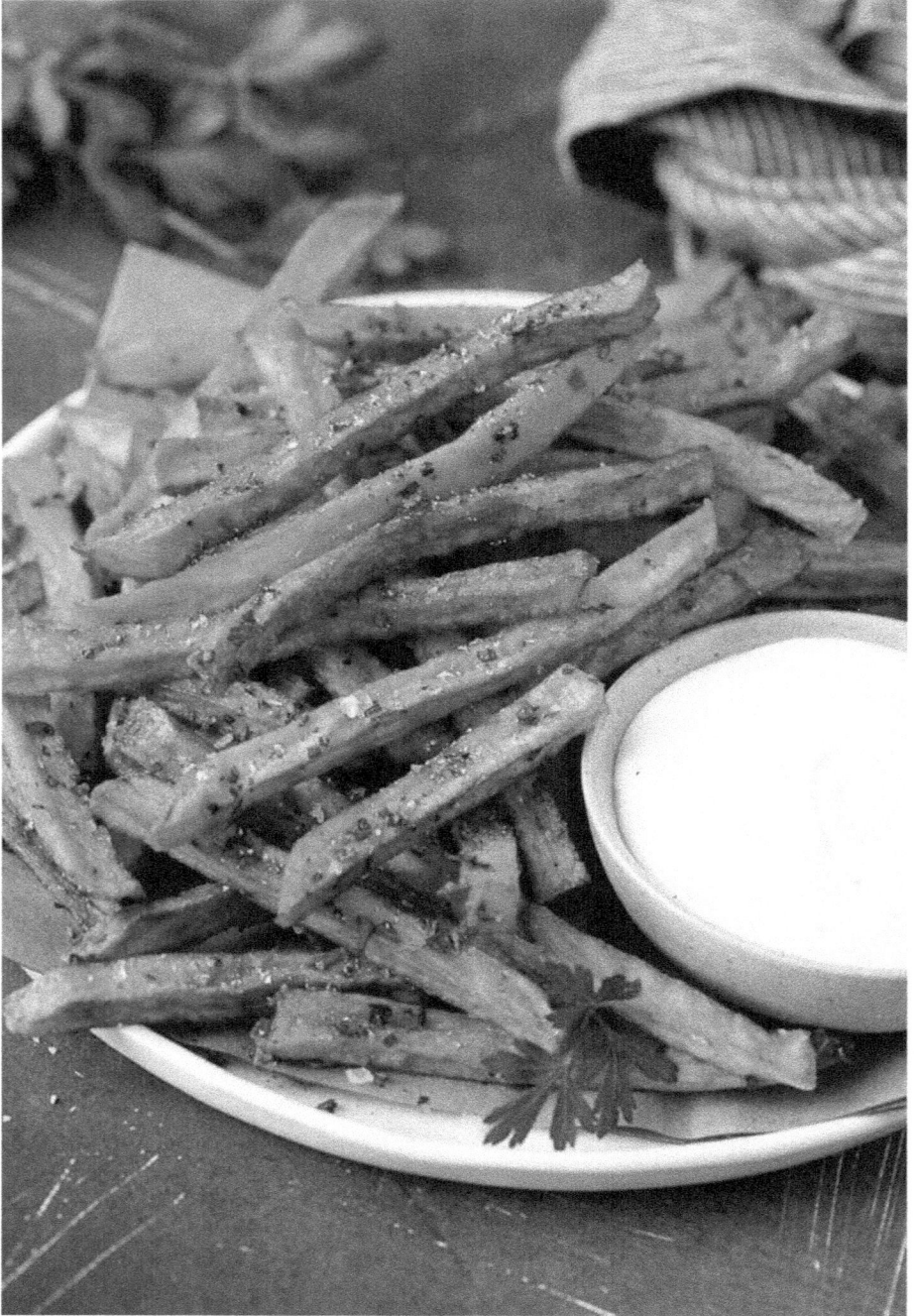

sources. Please consult a licensed professional before attempting any techniques outlined in this book.

By reading this document, the reader agrees that under no circumstances is the author responsible for any losses, direct or indirect, which are incurred as a result of the use of information contained within this document, including, but not limited to, — errors, omissions, or inaccuracies.

Table of Contents

Desserts Recipes

1   Keto Pecan Toffee Crunch

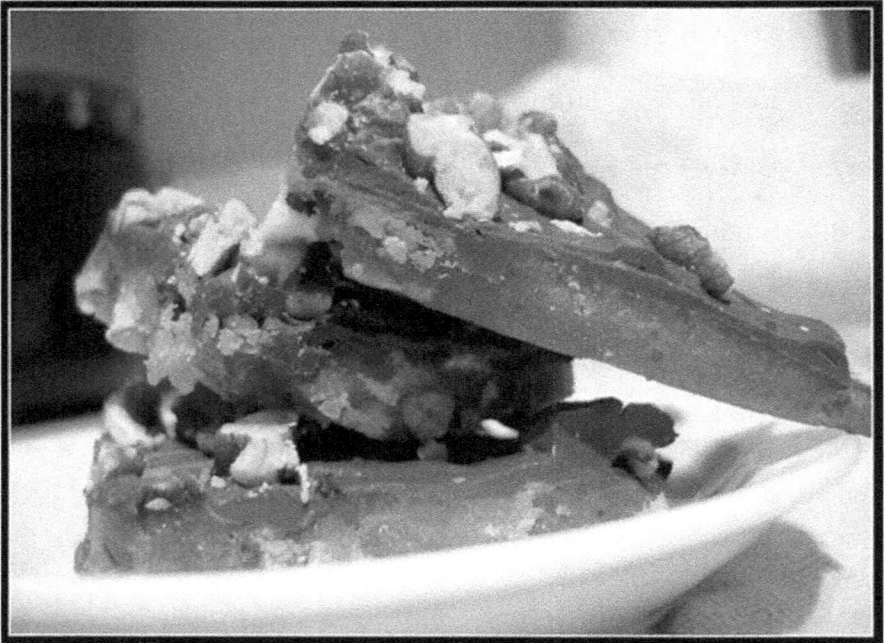

Servings: 12 | **Time:** 12 mins | **Difficulty:** Easy

Nutrients per serving: Calories: 660 kcal | Fat: 60g | Carbohydrates: 7g | Protein: 13g | Fiber: 7g

Ingredients

Pinch Himalayan or sea salt

4 cups pork rind pieces

½ tsp vanilla

½ cup butter

¼ cup finely chopped pecans

¼ cup + 2 Tbsp Lakanto Monkfruit (Golden) Sweetener

Method

1.   Line and set aside a sheet pan with the parchment. Place bits of pork rind in a medium bowl and place them aside.

2.   Combine the sweetener and butter in a tiny saucepan and melt on medium heat. Get it to a boil, continuously stirring. Switch the heat to medium-low and continue cooking for 5 minutes or so. To the butter mixture, add the pecans and finish cooking for a further 1-2 minutes or until the toasty pecans smell. Stir in the vanilla and salt and lift the butter mixture to the heat.

3.   Pour half of a butter mixture on the pork rinds or spoon it over and toss to cover it. Repeat with the mixture of butter that remains. You may also put the pork rinds on the pan and let

them cool to harden in the refrigerator. Store it in a sealed jar at room temperature and enjoy.

2   Jalapeno Mexican Fudge

Servings: 16-24 | **Time:** 45 mins | **Difficulty**: Easy

Nutrients per serving: Calories: 660 kcal | Fat: 60g | Carbohydrates: 7g | Protein: 13g | Fiber: 7g

Ingredients

1 jar (12oz) pickled, sliced jalapenos (drained)

1/2 Tsp. garlic powder

1/4 Tsp. onion powder

2 lbs Cheddar cheese (medium or mild), grated

2 lbs Monterrey Jack cheese, grated

7 oz cream or evaporated milk (Only a little over 3/4 cup)

7 whole eggs, beaten

Method

1.   Preheat the oven to 350 °F. Oiled a 9-to-13 pan gently.

2.   Range the sliced jalapenos in a single layer around the bottom of a plate. Test the heat with jalapenos. If you want less flame, you can use less or chop them up with jalapenos.

3.   Combine the shredded cheese, eggs, cream, garlic, and onion powder in a large mixing cup. Blend well.

4.   Pour the mixture of cheese over the jalapenos and scatter equally. Bake for about 45-55 minutes or until bubbly and golden brown.Until carving, cool for at least 20 minutes. Cool perfectly for optimum cutting results.

5.   Use 1lb of both Monterrey jack and cheddar, 3 beaten eggs, 6 tbsp of milk or cream, 1/8 tsp of powdered onion, and 1/4 tsp of garlic powder for a 9/9 pan. Similarly, cook the pan using half a packet of jalapenos. Then bake for 25-35 minutes.

3   Keto Banana Blueberry Muffins

Servings: 14 | **Time:** 30 mins | **Difficulty**: Easy

Nutrients per serving: Calories: 192 kcal | Fat: 16g | Carbohydrates: 6g | Protein: 6g | Fiber: 3g

Ingredients

¼ cup coconut flour

¼ cup sour cream

½ tsp salt

½ tsp. baking soda

1 cup diced raw zucchini

1 egg yolk

1 Tbsp. flaxseed meal

1 tsp. cinnamon

1 tsp. vanilla extract

2 cup almond flour

2 tsp. baking powder

2 tsp. quality banana extract, not imitation

3/4 cup frozen wild blueberries

5 eggs

6 Tbsp. butter melted

7 Tbsp. Lakanto Monkfruit (Golden) Sweetener, divided

Method

1.   Preheat the oven to 350°C. Using liners or mist to cover a muffin pan.

2.   In a shallow saucepan, pour 1 Tbsp. Of blueberries over medium heat. A pinch of salt and Lakanto. Bring the blend to a boil and drop the berries to a simmer, crushing them. Simmer that blueberry sauce until it thickens and the back of the spoon is coated for about 7 minutes.

3.   Combine the eggs, zucchini, egg yolk, and extracts in a blender and mix for about 10 seconds before the zucchini is pureed and light and fluffy.

4.   Combine the coconut flour and almond flour with the remaining sweetener, baking soda, salt, flax, and baking powder in a large bowl or the stand mixer bowl.

5.   Add the egg mixture to the dry ingredients, then mix with a paddle attachment at medium pace or by hand, once mixed,

scraping the sides at least once. Apply the sour cream and molten butter to the batter and stir until mixed.

6.   Spoon that thickened blueberries into the batter and whisk the blueberries softly over the batter, not perfectly rubbing it in.

7.   Spoon the batter uniformly into the already prepared muffin pan (approximately 3-4" full) and then bake at 350 F for 20 minutes or until baked.

8.   Bake until completed or for 20 minutes. Cool for 10 minutes in the pan and switch to the cooling rack to cool fully. Enjoy it with a coffee cup. These can be wrapped up and frozen for up to 3 days. And can be at room temperature for up to 5 days in the fridge.

4   Low Carb Shortbread Cookies

Servings: 24 | **Time:** 35 mins | **Difficulty**: Easy

Nutrients per serving: Calories: 62.2 kcal | Fat: 5.4g | Carbohydrates: 3.2g | Protein: 0.9g | Fiber: 0.3g

Ingredients

5 Tbsp. Monkfruit Sweetener

1 Tsp. Pure Vanilla Extract pinch of Salt

1/2 cup Ghee, at room temperature, the consistency of softened butter

2 1/2 Tsp. Pure Almond Extract

1/2 cup Tapioca Starch, plus 1 Tbsp. , 73g

3/4 cup Almond Flour, 73g

Method

1.   Preheat your oven to 350 ° F and line 2 parchment paper or silpats with baking sheets.

2.	Put the monk fruit in a SMALL food processor and process until perfect, and the powdered sugar consistency is around 3-4 minutes.

3.	In a large bowl, apply the monk fruit, with the ghee and all extracts. Using the electric hand mixer, run on high speed until very light yellow, around 3 minutes.

4.	Apply the flour, starch, and salt and beat for another 3 minutes again, stopping as needed to scrape the edges.

5.	Scoop back through the piping and pipe in 3⁄4-inch-high mounds on the prepared cookie sheet. These spread a lot, so leave space between them-I put 16 on one sheet of cookies. Do not down-press them.

6.	Bake for about 11-13 minutes before the edges just start to turn golden brown. Put the other sheet at room temperature before the first batch of cookies is finished if you can't get all sheets in at once.

7.	When baked, cool on the pan for about 10 minutes. Then turn a wire rack to cool fully.

5   Low Carb Corn Dog Muffins

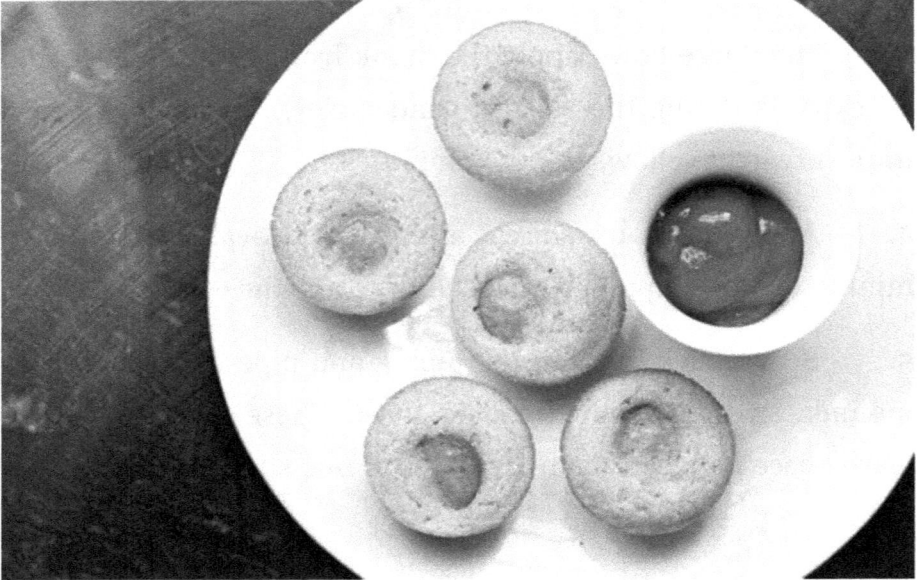

Servings: 6 | **Time:** 25 mins | **Difficulty:** Easy

Nutrients per serving: Calories: 274 kcal | Fat: 25g | Carbohydrates: 7g | Protein: 6g | Fiber: 3g

Ingredients

6 Tbsp. butter, melted

3 large eggs

2 Tbsp. sugar substitute

2 hot dogs

½ Tsp. salt

½ cup coconut flour

⅓ cup heavy cream

¼ Tsp. baking soda

Method

1.   Preheat the oven to 350°C. Using non-stick spray to spray a muffin pan.

2.   To a mixing cup, add the melted butter, milk, and eggs and whisk to blend.

3.   To mix, add the coconut flour, artificial sweetener, baking soda, and salt to the bowl and whisk well.

4.   Cut the hot dogs into little fragments and fold them into a mixture of cornbread. Spoon the mixture uniformly between the 6 muffin wells.

5.   Now Bake for about 15 minutes or until the muffin core comes out clean with a toothpick inserted into it. Until consuming, cool for 5 minutes.

6   Keto Buckeyes

Servings: 34 | **Time:** 1 hr 30 mins | **Difficulty**: Easy

Nutrients per serving: Calories: 164 kcal | Fat: 13g | Carbohydrates: 12g | Protein: 3g | Fiber: 2g

Ingredients

3½ cups confectioners swerve (if not keto, use powdered sugar)

3 cups lily's semisweet chocolate chips (if not keto, you can use chocolate wafers for easiest melting)

1 ⅓ cup all-natural peanut butter (for keto, use Just natural, if not making keto, use Jif)

1 Tsp. vanilla extract

1 Tbsp. coconut oil

½ cup salted butter softened

Method

1.   In a big bowl or mixer, combine the peanut sugar, butter, vanilla, and milk for about 30 seconds.

2.   In the cup, sift the swerve or powdered sugar and beat till smooth. For 30 minutes, cool the mixture in a refrigerator. Line a parchment paper baking sheet, slice out the peanut butter mixture with the medium cookie scoop and then roll it into balls.

3.   Put them on a cookie sheet and chill for 20 to 30 minutes in the fridge. Melt the chocolate and coconut oil in a large glass at 30-second intervals just before extracting the balls from the fridge, swirling each of them until fully melted.

4.   Spear the balls with a toothpick and dip them into the molten chocolate. Using a fork to help extract the ball from the toothpick and bring it back on the parchment pad.

5.   To lightly cover the toothpick opening, use your finger or the paring knife. Set until it hardens with the chocolate.

7 Keto Cookie Dough Ice Cream

Servings: 15 | **Time:** 1 hr 5 mins | **Difficulty**: Easy

Nutrients per serving: Calories: 660 kcal | Fat: 60g | Carbohydrates: 7g | Protein: 13g | Fiber: 7g

Ingredients

ICE CREAM:

2 large organic eggs

2 cups organic whipping cream

1 Tbsp vanilla extract

1/2 tsp fine sea salt

1/8 tsp almond extract (optional)

3/4 cup Lakanto Monk Fruit

1:1 Sweetener

2.5 cups organic whole milk

COOKIE DOUGH:

2 Tbsp milk

2 Tbsp Lakanto maple-flavored syrup

2 pinches sea salt

1/4 cup (50g) sugar-free chocolate chips

1 tsp vanilla extract

1 cup packed (150g) almond flour

Method

1.   Chill Fridge Ice Cream Canister (if directed by your ice cream machine instructions). To store ice cream in the fridge, you may want to cool the container you plan to use.

2.   Beat eggs with the whisk attachment on high in the stand mixer until foamy. Reduce the pace to low and include the sweetener progressively.

3.   Beat for 1 minute or before it thickens somewhat.

4.   Include the ice cream, sea salt, vanilla extract, and almond extract. Mix on medium until fully mixed.

5.   Pour in the ice cream canister and then pour the milk into it. If you double the formula and use a regular bucket ice cream

unit, fill the full filling line with milk (no more than 5 cups of milk).

6.   Or a spoon or a spatula, blend properly.

7.   In compliance with its directions, run the ice cream machine. Before operating the computer, this could involve cooling the liquid well. Simply search the manuals for your particular computer brand.

8.   Create cooked dough when churning the ice cream. In a medium-sized mixing bowl, combine all the ingredients except the chocolate chips. Stir well until it shapes dough. Stir in the chocolate chips and blend until blended. Form into small cookie dough balls by hands (approx 1cm in diameter). Apply a little extra almond flour if the dough is a little sticky. In the fridge, put the cookie dough balls (make sure they don't touch).

9.   Stir the cold cookie dough balls softly with a long spoon or spatula until the ice cream is done churning. At this point, your ice cream should have a soft serving consistency.

10.   To harden up the ice cream texture, put ice cream in a freezer in your storage vessel. Enjoy. Hold it in an airtight jar in the fridge.

8   Keto Buttermilk Biscuits

Servings: 6 | **Time:** 25 mins | **Difficulty:** Easy

Nutrients per serving: Calories: 660 kcal | Fat: 60g | Carbohydrates: 7g | Protein: 13g | Fiber: 7g

Ingredients

1/4 cup grass-fed collagen

1/4 cup reduced-fat buttermilk

1/2 tsp fine sea salt

2 cups packed (300g) finely ground blanched almond flour

2 tsp aluminum-free double-acting baking powder

2 Tbsp (28g) grass-fed butter

4 large egg whites

Method

1.   Preheat the oven to 375oF and cover the parchment paper with a baking sheet.

2.   In the medium-sized mixing dish, combine the dried ingredients.

3.   Using a cheese grater, grind in cold butter. Toss to merge those bits that have stayed together and split them up.

4.   Apply the buttermilk and the egg whites to the mixture and blend well.

5.   Make biscuits simply like drop biscuits. And then scoop the batter on the parchment paper (so you can form them by hand), or if you want good biscuits and don't mind the extra work, you need to spoon a mixture into a well-oiled cup and then softly press the batter down with your fingertips into the measuring cup and flip it.

6.   For 20-22 minutes, bake. This cooking time is for the biscuits with 1/3 cup of batter. If you've made the drop biscuits and smaller ones, you need to reduce the cooking time a little. When they have a good golden hue on them, the biscuits are finished.

7.   Leave the pan to cool for around 5 minutes, then switch off a cooling rack to stop cooling. Due to their soft texture, such biscuits are better if you let these cool for a minimum of 10 minutes before consuming them. For around 15-20 minutes, leave them.

9   Keto Crockpot Candy

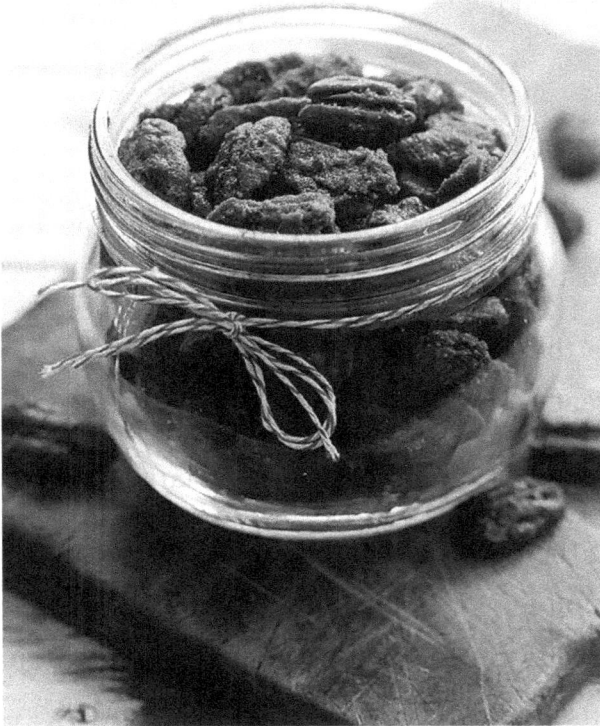

Servings: 24 | **Time:** 1 hr 3 mins | **Difficulty:** Easy

Nutrients per serving: Calories: 660 kcal | Fat: 60g | Carbohydrates: 7g | Protein: 13g | Fiber: 7g

Ingredients

2 1/2 cups (425g) Lily's Milk Chocolate Chips or Lily's Semi-Sweet Chocolate Chips

2 cups (280g) raw cashews

Decorative sprinkles,

Method

1.   In a small or a medium crockpot, place cashews in a layer. On top, pour the chocolate chips. You don't stir.

2.   Place the top of the lid and put it on low heat. Leave 1 hour for a seat.

3.   Line the parchment paper with a large baking sheet.

4.   Drop the cover after 1 hour and mix well. The chocolate should be molten, still not runny, but still a little dense. Rapidly scoop out candy on the parchment that is lined baking sheets using a soup spoon. Each candy should be around.

5.   Leave 5 minutes to cool, then decorate, if desired, with sprinkles.

6.   Place them in the refrigerator and leave for 45 minutes to harden. Take it from the fridge and enjoy it. Up to 1 week, you can store at room temperature in an airtight container.

10   Keto Cinnamon Roll Holes Donut

Servings: 24 | **Time:** 30 mins | **Difficulty**: Easy

Nutrients per serving: Calories: 660 kcal | Fat: 60g | Carbohydrates: 7g | Protein: 13g | Fiber: 7g

Ingredients

DONUT HOLE DOUGH:

1/4 cup (36g) of coconut flour

1 1/3 cup packed (200g) finely ground almond flour

1/2 tsp fine sea salt

2 Tbsp (28g) of Lakanto Monk Fruit (Golden) Sweetener

2 Tbsp (12g) grass-fed collagen

4 tsp aluminum-free double-acting baking powder

4 large eggs, beaten (about 210g)

FOR ROLLING THE DONUT HOLES:

3 Tbsp grass-fed butter or ghee, melted but not hot

1 Tbsp cinnamon

1/3 cup Lakanto Golden Monk Fruit Sweetener

CREAM CHEESE FROSTING:

1 tsp vanilla extract

1/3 cup cream cheese, softened

1/8 tsp sea salt

2 Tbsp grass-fed butter or ghee, softened

2 Tbsp powdered erythritol or Lakanto Golden Coconut milk or almond milk to thin

Method

1.	Preheat the oven to 3500°F/1770°C and cover the parchment paper with a baking sheet.

2.	Just make the dough. Combine the dried ingredients in a large mixing bowl and blend well. Add the eggs and blend well until they form a dough. The dough can hold well together, but it's always going to be sort of wet, not dry.

3.	"Make "sugar with cinnamon. Mix the cinnamon and the 1/3 cup of Lakanto Golden in a small bowl or plate to produce the cinnamon sugar. Through a small dish, pour molten butter.

4.　　Shape the balls into a pastry. Scoop out rounded tbsp of dough using a tbsp measurement and roll with your hands to make balls. Roll throughout the butter to coat as you shape each ball, then roll in cinnamon sugar. Place it on a baking sheet lined with parchment and begin with the remaining dough.

5.　　For 15 minutes, roast them. Create the frosting before icing the donut holes. Whip the melted butter & cream cheese together for a few minutes, using a stand mixer or a hand mixer. Add erythritol, sea salt powder, vanilla, and whip for another few minutes until soft and light. To thin to the desired consistency, blend in coconut or almond milk as needed. Drizzle and serve with frosting.

11   Low Carb Pumpkin Spice Meriques

Servings: 55 cookies | **Time:** 25 mins | **Difficulty**: Easy

Nutrients per serving: Calories: 2 kcal | Fat: 1g | Carbohydrates: 2g | Protein: 1g | Fiber: 1g

Ingredients

4 large egg whites

2 tsp. pumpkin pie spice, no sugar added

1/2 tsp. cream of tartar

3/4 cup erythritol, powdered in a blender

Method

1.   Preheat the oven to 200 ºF.

2.   Beat the whites of the egg until they are almost stiff.

3.   Fold and finish pounding before you have stiff peaks in the erythritol and pumpkin pie spice.

4.   Place on a parchment-lined baking sheet with dollops of whipped egg. Use your size judgment.

5.   With the oven door partly open, bake for 2 1/2 to 3 hours. By inserting a wooden spoon between the door and the oven, this can be accomplished.

12 Keto Sugar-Free Lemon Meringue Pie

Servings: 8 | **Time**: 3 hrs 45 mins | **Difficulty**: Easy

Nutrients per serving: Calories: 199 kcal | Fat: 16g | Carbohydrates: 14g | Protein: 7g | Fiber: 3g

Ingredients

1 batch of low carb pie crust Keto Lemon Curd

3/4 cup lemon juice

3 large eggs yolk

1/8 Tsp. stevia powder

1/3 cup powdered erythritol

1 Tbsp. lemon zest

1 Tbsp. arrowroot powder Meringue Topping

3 egg whites

1/2 Tsp. cream of tartar

Method

1.   As per directions, prepare the low carb crust. Press the dough into a tart pan or an oiled pastry—Bake for 15 minutes at 325 °F.

2.   Prepare a lemon curd by putting a small pot on medium-low flame. Apply the juice of the lemon, then heat until lukewarm.

3.   Whisk together the egg yolks, arrowroot powder, powdered erythritol, stevia powder, and the lemon zest in a medium sized-mixing bowl. To temper the eggs, whisk the mild hot lemon juice in the egg mixture and continue whisking until whole juice is poured.

4.   Return the lemon curd to the pot on its whole back and heat on medium heat, stirring at a medium pace. (NOTE: Steady stirring is the secret to a good custard. Not as easy as scrambled eggs, but not so sluggish that things burst or boil.)

5.   Continue to stir before the gravy thickens (about 3-5 minutes). Pour the lemon curd in the prepared pie crust until thickened and put uncovered for at least 2 hours in the fridge to stiffen and cool.

6.   In a medium bowl with tartar cream, make your meringue top by beating egg whites until egg whites become glossy and form firm peaks.

7.   To build peaks for browning, spoon meringue on top of a pie dab. Set for a few minutes under a high- heat broiler, regularly rotating to cook uniformly. Look carefully if you want to toast the meringue, but not roast it. Once it achieves the quality, you expect. Leave it to cool for another hour in the refrigerator before serving.

13   Keto Chocolate Fudge

Servings: 30 | **Time:** 40 mins | **Difficulty**: Easy

Nutrients per serving: Calories: 143 kcal | Fat: 12g | Carbohydrates: 14g | Protein: 2g | Fiber: 3g

Ingredients

4 Tbsp. butter

3 cups low carb chocolate chips

2 Tsp. xanthan gum

2 Tbsp. monk fruit sweetener

1 Tsp. vanilla extract

1 1/2 cups heavy whipping cream

Method

1.   In a small pot, pour heavy whipping cream and bring to medium heat to boil. Reduce to simmer for about 30 minutes until boiling. To avoid the development of skin, whisk or stir regularly.

2. Apply the vanilla, butter, and sugar at room temperature to the simmering cream and then whisk until well mixed.

3. Include the xanthan gum and mix thoroughly so that no clumps are present.

4. Remove from the heat and add the chocolate chips immediately, whisking until thoroughly mixed. After several minutes of whisking, if not smooth, adjust to low heat and whisk until it is smooth.

5. In an oiled or parchment-lined 6x9 or 8x8 pan/casserole dish, pour immediately.

6. Chill uncovered for at least 4 hours in a refrigerator, overnight if feasible.

7. Cut between parchment paper sheets for gifting and serving or packaging.

14   Low Carb Chocolate Cake

Servings: 8 | **Time:** 45 mins | **Difficulty**: Easy

Nutrients per serving: Calories: 237 kcal | Fat: 10g | Carbohydrates: 41g | Protein: 4g | Fiber: 3g

Ingredients

3 tbsp butter unsalted and melted

2 eggs at room temperature

2 cups low carb vanilla frosting

1/4 tsp salt

1/4 cup powdered sweetener

1/4 cup brown sugar alternative

1/2 tsp vanilla extract

1/2 Tsp. baking soda

1/2 cup unsweetened cocoa powder

1/2 cup unsweetened almond milk

1/2 cup coconut flour

1 tsp apple cider vinegar

1 Tsp. baking powder

Method

1.   Preheat the oven to 350 °F

2.   Pre-oiled two pans of the 6-inch round cake.

3.   Mix the almond milk and the apple cider vinegar in a shallow bowl.

4.   Mix the dry ingredients in a big bowl: sweetener, almond flour, baking soda, coconut flour, salt, baking powder, and brown sugar. Build a well for the wet ingredients in the middle.

5.   Add the vanilla powder, sugar, and eggs and blend to combine. Pour the combination of milk in and blend well.

6.   Distribute the cake batter uniformly into your rectangular cake pans. Tap pans to disperse the cake mixture thinly around the pan on a flat surface to eliminate excess air.

7.   Now Bake for 20 to 25 minutes before it comes out clean when the toothpick is inserted. Until frosting, cause your cake to completely cool.

15 Keto Chocolate Cheesecake Mousse

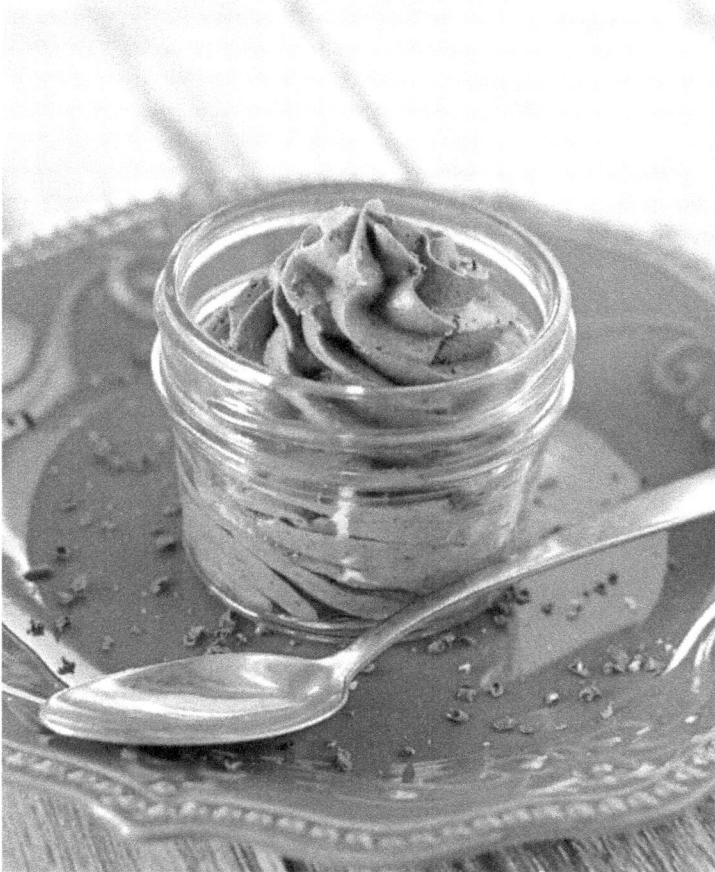

Servings: 5 | **Time:** 10 mins | **Difficulty**: Easy

Nutrients per serving: Calories: 329 kcal | Fat: 34g | Carbohydrates: 15g | Protein: 5g | Fiber: 1g

Ingredients

1/4 cup powdered erythritol

1/4 cup cocoa powder

1 cup heavy whipping cream

1 cup cream cheese

Method

1.   Add all of the ingredients to a big bowl and use a hand mixer to mix the ingredients for 2 minutes. Scrape the bowl's sides off. Mix for a further 3 minutes until the stiff peaks are produced, and the mixture is dense and creamy.

2.   To taste, apply additional sweeteners. In the airtight container, store your chocolate whipped cream in the refrigerator for 3 days.

16 Low Carb Chocolate Cauldron Cupcakes

Servings: 6 | **Time:** 40 mins | **Difficulty**: Easy

Nutrients per serving: Calories: 320 kcal | Fat: 30g | Carbohydrates: 34g | Protein: 8g | Fiber: 5g

Ingredients

Low Carb Chocolate Cupcake:

3/4 cup almond flour

3 large whole eggs

1/4 cup unsweetened cocoa powder

1/2 cup grapeseed oil

1/2 cup erythritol

1 tsp. pure vanilla extract

1 tbsp of baking powder

Chocolate Frosting:

1/2 cup coconut fat

1/4 cup erythritol

1/4 cup unsweetened cocoa powder

Method

1.   Wash the cauldrons and, if used, dry them. Place them on a parchment-lined cookie sheet. Otherwise, line the muffin tins with the liners you've picked.

2.   Preheat a 350 F microwave. Combine the cupcake items in a medium mixing dish, swirling well to mix.

3.   In the cauldrons or the cupcake liners, part the batter out. Bake for 20-30 minutes, roughly.

.Notice that in a convection oven. That can be done with a cake tester, which pulls out clean when poked.

4.   When cupcakes are in the oven, prepare the frosting by combining the frosting products in a small-medium mixing bowl with the electric beater—store until available to use in the refrigerator.

5.   Cool them fully before top with the frosting when the cupcakes are completed baked. Serving and enjoying.

17   Keto Pound Cake

Servings: 10 | **Time:** 1 hr 5 mins | **Difficulty:** Easy

Nutrients per serving: Calories: 175 kcal | Fat: 16g | Carbohydrates: 23g | Protein: 5g | Fiber: 1g

Ingredients

4 eggs

1/4 cup cream cheese

1/4 cup butter

1/2 cup sour cream

1 Tsp. vanilla extract

1 Tsp. baking powder

1 Tbsp. coconut flour

1 cup monk fruit sweetener

1 cup almond flour

Method

1.   Preheat the oven to 350 Fahrenheit

2.   By oiling with butter and then lining with parchment paper, prepare the 9-inch flat bottom plate.

3.   Whisk the almond flour, baking powder, and coconut flour together in a big dish.

4.   Add butter and cream cheese in a different dish. Microwave on high for about 30 seconds, whisk and microwave for additional 30 seconds if desired before butter and the cream cheese melts together. Stir in the vanilla extract, sweetener, and sour cream. Then mix properly.

5.   Pour the cream cheese butter mixture into a dry mixture. Stir once mixed properly. Apply the eggs to the batter when well mixed, one at a time.

6.   Pour the batter into the dish. Bake for 55 minutes or until it comes out clean with a toothpick.

7.   In a bundt pan, allow the cake to cool entirely; we've found it's best to let it cool completely for hours before it reaches room temperature (just like a cheesecake)

8.   Serve with whipped cream and fresh strawberries.

18   Low Carb Mock Apple Pie

Servings: 8 | **Time:** 1 hr | **Difficulty**: Easy

Nutrients per serving: Calories: 190 kcal | Fat: 16g | Carbohydrates: 20g | Protein: 6g | Fiber: 5g

Ingredients

3 cups chopped zucchini, peeled and finely chopped

1/8 tsp ground allspice

1/2 tsp ground nutmeg

1/2 tsp ground cardamom

1/2 cup monk fruit sweetener (or another low carb granular sweetener)

1 tsp. pure liquid stevia

1 tbsp lemon juice

1 tbsp butter, chopped

1 batch low carb pie crust

1 1/2 tsp ground cinnamon

Method

1.	Have the pie crust primed, but under-cook it (for almost 5-7 minutes).

2.	Mix all the ingredients in a mixing bowl and stir well to cover the zucchini evenly with spices and sweetener.

3.	For about 40 minutes or until a zucchini cooked to your taste, pour a zucchini into pie crust, wrap loosely with foil, and bake.

4.	Until serving, cool perfectly.

5.	Remember that this is good with low carbohydrate whipped cream

19   Keto Ice Cream

Servings: 4 | **Time:** 6 hrs 45 mins | **Difficulty**: Easy

Nutrients per serving: Calories: 439 kcal | Fat: 45g | Carbohydrates: 13g | Protein: 5g | Fiber: 1g

Ingredients

4 egg yolks, beaten

1 Tsp. vanilla extract

1/2 cup low carb syrup

1 3/4 cup heavy cream

Method

1.   Whip the heavy cream with the hand mixer in a large bowl until it forms stiff peaks. Only put aside.

2.   In a small dish, heat the low-carb syrup until it boils.

3.   Meanwhile, add a big glass bowl of pounded egg yolks. Slowly drizzle the pounded egg yolks with sweet syrup until you have a pale and cream combination. Add an extract of vanilla.

4.   Fold in the egg mixture with the whipped cream.

5.   In a loaf tin, pour the mixture and cover it with plastic wrap. Put in the freezer and leave to set for at least 4-6 hours.

20 Low Carb Chocolate Fondue

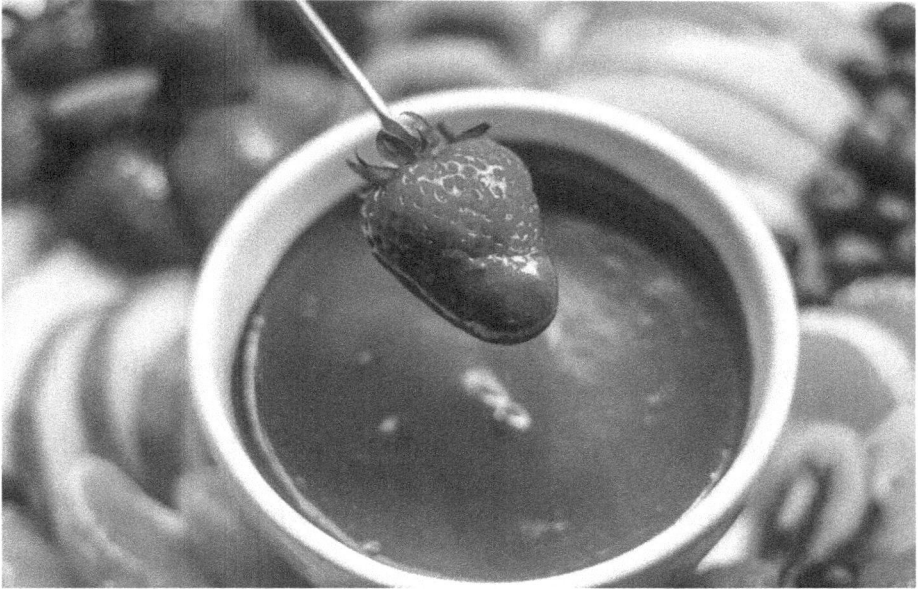

Servings: 7 | **Time:** 1 hr 5 mins | **Difficulty**: Easy

Nutrients per serving: Calories: 194 kcal | Fat: 19g | Carbohydrates: 21g | Protein: 3g | Fiber: 4g

Ingredients

1 cup coconut milk (canned, full fat)

1 oz. brandy

1/2 cup erythritol (or another low carb granular sweetener)

1/4 tsp. pure liquid stevia

6 oz. unsweetened chocolate

Method

1.   In a small and 1 quart slow cooker, combine all ingredients and mix to combine.

2.   Switch the low setting slow cooker and cover with the lid.

3.   Cook for approx 1 hour or until it's melted with chocolate.

4.   To mix everything in the pot, stir or whisk.

5.   Switch the temp to "Keep Warm" and serve with low carb fruits such as raspberries or blueberries and strawberries from the crock.

6.   Don't miss the forks of fondue

Snack

21 Instant Pot Turnip Greens & Collard Greens

Servings: 6 | **Time**: 20 mins | **Difficulty**: Easy

Nutrients per serving: Calories: 256 kcal | Fat: 23g | Carbohydrates: 8g | Protein: 3g | Fiber: 3g

Ingredients

20 oz. Turnip greens or collard greens (stem removed and roughly chopped)

1 cup Chicken broth

½ cup Onion, diced

2 tbsp Vinegar

Salt and pepper to taste

6 oz. Salt pork (diced into about 1/4-inch pieces)

Method

1.   Set the Instant pot to saute, add pork or bacon salt and onions, and cook until the pork is crisp and the onions become softened.

2.   Pour the chicken broth into a pot and deglaze the pan's bottle to ensure the browned bits get up. To stop the saute feature, click cancel.

3.   In the greens, add some vinegar and the package so that the pot is around 2/3 of the way finished.

4.   Lock the lid and turn the valve to the SEALING position. For 10 minutes, set to high Intensity.

5.   When the timer goes off, adjust the valve to Ventilation and let all the air out by rapidly opening it.

6.   To blend it, remove the lid, swirl the pot's contents, and apply salt and black pepper.

22   Keto Avocado Coleslaw

Servings: 8 | **Time**: 10 mins | **Difficulty**: Easy

Nutrients per serving: Calories: 123 kcal | Fat: 10g | Carbohydrates: 8g | Protein: 2g | Fiber: 4g

Ingredients

1/2 cup Sour Cream

1/2 tsp salt

16 oz. Coleslaw mix (or shredded cabbage)

2 Avocado

3-4 tbsp Lime Juice (more to taste)

Method

1.   Stir mixture into coleslaw.

2.   Mash avocado with sour cream, lime juice, and salt.

3.   Keep refrigerated until you are ready to serve.

23 Buffalo Chicken Jalapeño Poppers

Servings: 8 | **Time:** 50 mins | **Difficulty:** Easy

Nutrients per serving: Calories: 408 kcal | Fat: 33g | Carbohydrates: 4g | Protein: 21g

Ingredients

8 oz. Cream Cheese, softened

3 tbsp Ranch Dressing

2 Chicken Breasts (approximately 12 oz.)

1/2 cup Frank's Red Hot sauce

1/2 cup Cheddar Cheese, (shredded)

Buffalo Chicken Jalapeño Poppers (Make Almost 30 Poppers)

16-20 Jalapeños, halved

16-20 Strips Bacon Buffalo Chicken Dip,

Method

Buffalo Chicken Dip:

1.   Boil the water.

2.   For 15 minutes, or when cooked through, put the chicken breasts in the boiling water.

3.   Remove the chicken breasts and insert them directly in the mixing bowl of the stand mixer. (You should use the fork to shred a chicken by hand if you do not have a stand mixer.)

4.   Turn the mixer to medium for about 1-2 minutes or until the chicken is entirely shredded using a dough hook. To make sure all the chicken becomes shredded, stir once or twice.

5.   Transfer the chicken to the softened cream cheese and mix it thoroughly.

6.   Apply the hot sauce and thoroughly mix.

7.   Include the ranch and shredded cheese and mix thoroughly.

Buffalo Chicken Jalapeño Poppers:

1.   Preheat the oven to 400° F.

2.   Cook bacon partly, making it partly crisp but still flexible enough to coil around the poppers.

3.   With a heaping tbsp of buffalo chicken sauce, stuff the jalapeno halves with it.

4.   Wrap a slice of bacon for each jalapeño popper.

5.   On a baking sheet, place the stuffed poppers.

6.   Bake until the jalapeños are softened, and the bacon is crispy in the oven. 20 minutes roughly.

24   Low Carb Big Mac Bites

Servings: 16 | **Time:** 35 mins | **Difficulty:** Easy

Nutrients per serving: Calories: 182 kcal | Fat: 12g | Carbohydrates: 1g | Protein: 10g

Ingredients

¼ cup Onion, finely diced

1 tsp salt

1.5 lb Ground beef

16 slices Dill Pickle

4 slices American Cheese Lettuce

SECRET SAUCE

1 tsp Garlic powder

1 tsp Onion powder

1 tsp Paprika

1 tsp White wine vinegar

1/2 cup Mayonnaise

2 tbsp yellow mustard

4 tbsp Dill pickle relish

Method

1.   Preheat the oven to 400°F.

2.   Mix the onions, ground beef, and salt in a large dish. Mix when mixed thoroughly.

3.   Roll the beef into balls of 1.5 oz.. To make the mini burger patty, press every one slightly down to flatten it and put it on the lined baking sheet.

4.   Now Bake for 15 minutes or until fully baked at 400 °F.

5.   When cooking burgers, add all the secret sauce components to a bowl and mix to blend.

6.   Switch off the oven when the burgers baking finished and remove them—Pat off the extra oil.

7.   Cut four squares of each cheese slice and put a square on each mini-patty. Place the cheese back in the oven and let it melt.

8.   Place a few lettuces (squares) and a pickle slice on top of each meatball, and drive a skewer through it. Serve or have the special sauce.

25 Ranch Baked Pork Chops

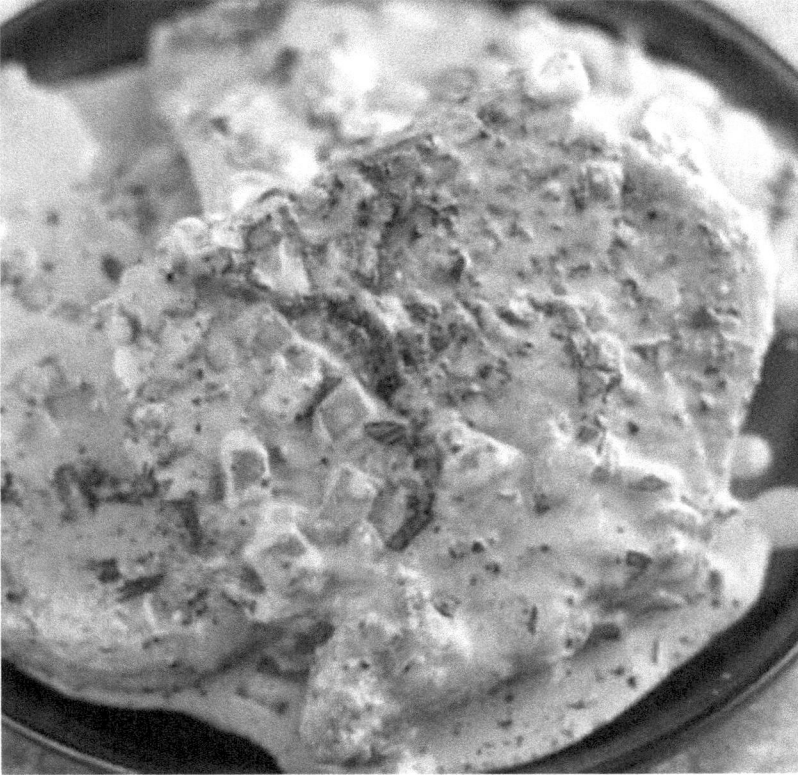

Servings: 4 | **Time:** 35 mins | **Difficulty:** Easy

Nutrients per serving: Calories: 252 kcal | Fat: 9g | Carbohydrates: 7g | Protein: 32g

Ingredients

4 Pork Chops,

1 inch thick 2 tsp Dried Parsley

2 tsp Garlic Powder

2 tsp Paprika

1 tsp Dried Dill Weed

1 tsp Dried Minced Onions

1 tsp Sea Salt

½ tsp Dried Chives

½ tsp Onion Powder

1/2 tsp Ground Black Pepper

1/4 cup Dry Buttermilk Powder

Method

1.   Preheat the oven to 400°F.

2.   To make the ranch seasoning, add all the dry ingredients in the bowl and blend thoroughly.

3.   In the ranch seasoning, dip each pork chop, turning it over when it is thoroughly coated. Before lying on a baking sheet, shake off the residue.

4.   In the oven, put the pork chops and bake for 15 to 25 minutes. When it touches an internal temperature of 145 °F, the pork chop is cooked.

5.   Until eating, let the pork chops rest for about 5 minutes.

26　Low Carb Nachos

Servings: 8 | **Time:** 35 mins | **Difficulty**: Easy

Nutrients per serving: Calories: 227 kcal | Fat: 14g | Carbohydrates: 6g | Protein: 18g | Fiber: 1g

Ingredients

Toppings such as avocado, sour cream, tomatoes,

8 oz Cheddar Cheese (shredded)

20 Mini Sweet Peppers (halved and seeded)

2 tbsp Chili Powder

1/2 tsp salt

1 tbsp Cumin

1 lb Ground Beef, chicken, steak, or pork, cooked

1 Jalapeno, sliced

Method

1.   Cook your favorite meat in a skillet, adding cumin, chili powder, and salt. On a sheet plate, put the mini sweet pepper halves.

2.   Sprinkle the cooked meat over the mini peppers and hold it in peppers to spill into the pan. Cover the mini peppers with jalapeno slices and shredded cheese.

3.   Put in a BROIL-set oven for about 5-6 minutes or when the cheese is completely melted.

4.   Apply some low carb toppings you need for the nacho.

27　Air Fryer Low Carb Mozzarella Sticks

Servings: 6 | **Time:** 20 mins | **Difficulty**: Easy

Nutrients per serving: Calories: 267 kcal | Fat: 20g | Carbohydrates: 4g | Protein: 18g | Fiber: 1g

Ingredients

1 tsp Italian seasoning

1/2 cup Almond flour

1/2 cup Parmesan cheese (the powdered form)

1/2 tsp Garlic Salt

12 Mozzarella sticks, string cheese (cut in half)

2 large eggs, beaten

Method

1.　Mix the almond flour, Italian seasoning, parmesan cheese, and garlic salt in a dish. Whisk the eggs together in a separate dish.

2.   Coat the mozzarella stick halves in your egg one at a time and then toss throughout the coating combination. Please place them in a suitable jar.

3.   Place parchment paper among the mozzarella sticks layers if you need to make more than 1 sheet. Freeze for 30 minutes the sticks of mozzarella

4.   Remove it from the freezer and placed it in the Philips AirFryer.

5.   Adjust to 400 °F for 5 minutes and cook.

6.   Open the air fryer and then let for 1 min before moving to a plate of low carbohydrate mozzarella sticks.

28 Crab Cakes With Roasted Red Pepper Sauce

Servings: 8 | **Time:** 40 mins | **Difficulty**: Easy

Nutrients per serving: Calories: 65 kcal | Fat: 4g | Carbohydrates: 4g | Protein: 6g

Ingredients

2 tsp Old Bay seasoning

2 tsp dijon mustard

2 Tbsp parsley, chopped

2 Tbsp coconut oil

1.5 Tbsp coconut flour

1 Tbsp fresh lemon juice

1 egg, beaten

1 cup lump crab meat

Method

1.   1.Pick the crab carefully to ensure the absence of shells or the cartilage in meat and add it to a small bowl. Mix the lemon juice, egg, and dijon mustard in another small cup, blending until smooth.

2.   Mix the parsley, old bay, and coconut flour in a third dish, stirring thoroughly. Add the mixture of eggs to the crab softly, folding when mixed. Then apply to the crab mixture the dry ingredients and gently blend in. Try not to cut up the crab bits or shred them too far.

3.   Heat the coconut oil in a nonstick saute pan over medium heat. Create 8 small cakes and carefully put them in the hot oil. Cook on either side for around 2-3 minutes, or until golden brown. Move to a plate lined with paper towels from the dish.

4.   Sprinkle with kosher salt and serve with the Roasted Red Pepper Sauce and half squeeze a fresh lemon over it.

29 Low Carb Taco Bites

Servings: 30 | **Time:** 1 hr | **Difficulty:** Easy

Nutrients per serving: Calories: 73 kcal | Fat: 5g | Carbohydrates: 1g | Protein: 4g

Ingredients

Pico de Gallo for garnish

8 tsp Sour Cream for garnish

2 tbsp Cumin

2 tbsp Chili Powder

2 cup Packaged Shredded Cheddar Cheese

1 tsp salt + more to taste

1 lb Ground Beef

Method

1.   Preheat the oven to 350 °F. Place 1 tbsp pile of cheese 2 inches apart on the baking sheet lined with a silicone or mat parchment paper

2.   Place the baking sheet in an oven and bake until the edges of cheese become brown, or for 5-7 minutes.

3.   Let that cheese cool for 1 min, then pick it up and press it down into a mini muffin tin cup to shape a cup.

4.   Let the cheese fully cool, and then cut it.

5.   As you begin to bake the cheese and make your cups, over medium-high heat heating, put the ground beef in the skillet until it is fully cooked.

6.   Drain the beef from the fat and then add 1/4 c of water and the spices.

7.   Stir once mixed, then add some more salt to taste and boil for 5 minutes.

8.   For cheese cups, substitute meat and finish each with 1/4 tsp of sour cream. If you like, you can also include fresh pico de gallo as well.

30 Bacon Cheese Balls

Servings: 24 | **Time**: 10 mins | **Difficulty**: Easy

Nutrients per serving: Calories: 89 kcal | Fat: 8g | Carbohydrates: 1g | Protein: 2g

Ingredients

10 slices bacon (finely chopped)

4 oz. Cheddar cheese (shredded)

4 oz. Salted Almonds (chopped)

8 oz. Cream cheese

Method

1.   In a dish, mix the first 3 ingredients.

2.   Roll the cheese mixture in 1-inch balls and roll and widen the ends slightly to gently mold them in an oval shape.

3.   Roll out the sliced almonds with the mini cubes.

31   Shrimp Cocktail Deviled Eggs

Servings: 12 | **Time:** 30 mins | **Difficulty:** Easy

Nutrients per serving: Calories: 142 kcal | Fat: 11g | Carbohydrates: 1g | Protein: 8g

Ingredients

1 1/2 tsp Horseradish

1/2 cup Mayonnaise

12 eggs, hard-boiled & peeled

24 Shrimp, steamed

3 tbsp Ketchup

Paprika for garnish

Salt to taste

Method

1.   Put the eggs in half and place the yolks in a different bowl to remove them.

2.   Apply the yolks to the horseradish, mayonnaise, ketchup, and salt and mix until creamy.

3.   In a piping bag, put the yolk mixture and pipe in the egg halves.

4.   Place a shrimp over each shell. Garnish with Paprika.

32 Shrimp Pil Pil

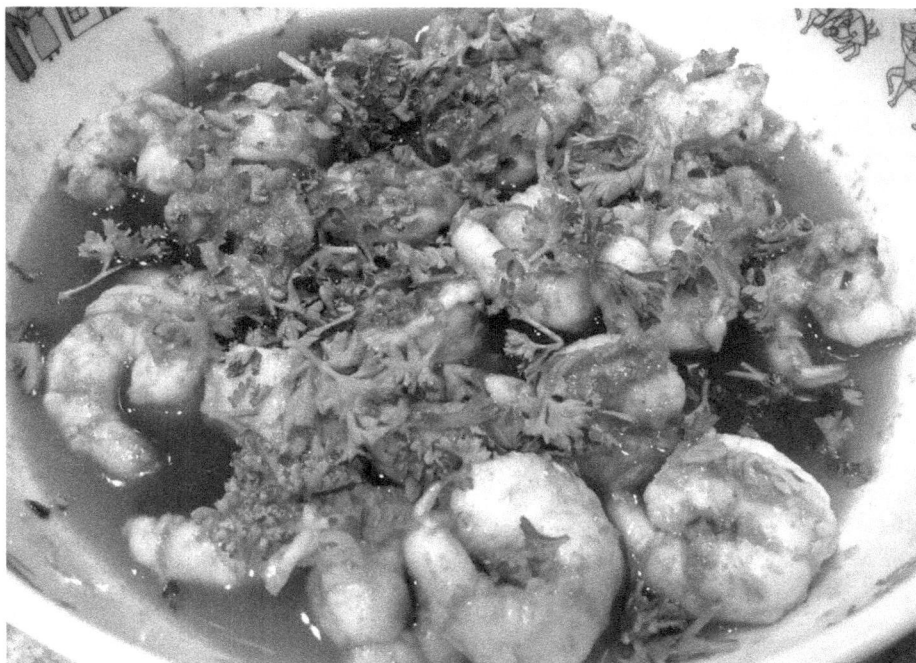

Servings: 8 | **Time:** 10 mins | **Difficulty**: Easy

Nutrients per serving: Calories: 275 kcal | Fat: 25g | Carbohydrates: 2g | Protein: 14g | Fiber: 2g

Ingredients

1 lb Shrimp, large (around 30 shrimp)

5 tbsp Butter

4 tbsp Tabasco

1 tbsp Spanish paprika

1 tsp Salt

2/3 c Olive oil

Method

1. Mix in the olive oil, sugar, Tabasco, paprika, and salt.

2. Place each ramekin with 3-4 shrimp and many slices of garlic.

3. Until the shrimp is partially covered, add the sauce in.

4. Put the ramekins on the baking sheet and broil them for 4-5 minutes in the oven or until the shrimp's oil bubbles and the shrimp become pink.

5. Remove from the oven and serve when hot.

33 Easy Guacamole

Servings: 12 | **Time**: 40 mins | **Difficulty**: Easy

Nutrients per serving: Calories: 178 kcal | Fat: 15g | Carbohydrates: 14g | Protein: 3g | Fiber: 8g

Ingredients

1 Roma or vine tomato

1/4 cup chopped fresh cilantro

1/4 cup chopped red onion

1-2 jalapeño or serrano chilis

2 ripe avocados

2-3 limes sea salt

Method

1.   Peel and pit the avocado and cut the onion thinly, and add it to a dish. Mush up the entire avocado with a fork.

2.   Drop the seeds and the liquid, wash and slice the tomato into half, then dice just the flesh and return it to the cup.

3.   Wash and spin fresh cilantro dry and cut when you have around 1/4 cup of cilantro chopped and return it to the dish.

4.   Season with lime juice and sea salt, stir it together well, and serve

5.   Add freshly chopped chili to the hot guacamole, too.

34   Keto Parmesan Roasted Broccoli

Servings: 5 | **Time:** 30 mins | **Difficulty**: Easy

Nutrients per serving: Calories: 157 kcal | Fat: 13.8g | Carbohydrates: 4.5g | Protein: 5.5g | Fiber: 2.2g

Ingredients

3 Tbsp. salted butter, melted

2 Tbsp. avocado oil

1/3 cup grated Parmesan cheese

1/2 tsp. salt

1/2 tsp. garlic powder

1 lb fresh broccoli florets

1 1/2 tsp. lemon pepper

Method

1.   Line and set aside a sheet pan with the parchment. Preheat the oven to 400°F.

2.   Place the florets of the broccoli in a wide dish. Mix the melted butter, avocado oil, garlic powder, lemon pepper, and salt in a separate bowl and mix.

3.   Drizzle over the broccoli with the butter mixture and toss to mix. Sprinkle the broccoli with parmesan and flip to cover it.

4.   On the ready sheet pan, put the broccoli into a single layer. Bake for about 20-25 minutes or until it is soft and golden brown.

35 Spicy Sautéed Mushrooms with Anchovy

Servings: 4 | **Time**: 20 mins | **Difficulty**: Easy

Nutrients per serving: Calories: 111 kcal | Fat: 8g | Carbohydrates: 9g | Protein: 3g | Fiber: 3g

Ingredients

Juice from 1 lemon optional

3 garlic cloves minced

2 tbsp butter or ghee

2 medium anchovy fillets

1 lb mixed mushrooms

¼ tsp red pepper flakes

Method

1.   Heat butter over medium-high heat in a large skillet. Apply the pepper flakes, anchovies, and garlic, as the butter melts and the foam subsides and cooked, splitting the anchovy

fillets with a wooden spoon before the mixture is fragrant (approx 1 minute).

2.   Include the mushrooms and cook for about 12 minutes, stirring regularly, until the mushrooms' liquid disappears and the mushrooms are finely browned. Season to taste with salt, squeeze one lemon juice (if used), and serve immediately.

36   Keto Cheese Crackers

Servings: 11 | **Time:** 30 mins | **Difficulty**: Easy

Nutrients per serving: Calories: 183 kcal | Fat: 17g | Carbohydrates: 4g | Protein: 6g | Fiber: 2g

Ingredients

5 Tbsp. butter salted & softened

4 oz. Pepper Jack cheese shredded

2 Tbsp. coconut flour

1 oz cream cheese softened

1 cup almond flour

¼ tsp. Salt

¼ tsp. Onion powder

¼ tsp. Garlic powder

¼ tsp. cumin

¼ cup finely chopped pecans

Method

1.   Cream together the butter and cream cheese in the tank of the stand mixer. Apply the melted cheese and blend until mixed properly. Add the 6 ingredients, then continue blending. Stir the chopped pecans together.

2.   Layer dough in plastic wrap and shape around 2 ½ inches thick into a roll. Tightly cover-up and cool or freeze until solid.

3.   Cut the chilled dough into ¼' thick slices and put on a sheet pan lined with parchment. Bake for 20-25 minutes at 300 °F or until softly golden brown. Before withdrawing, cool crackers entirely in pots.

37   Cheesy Squash Bites

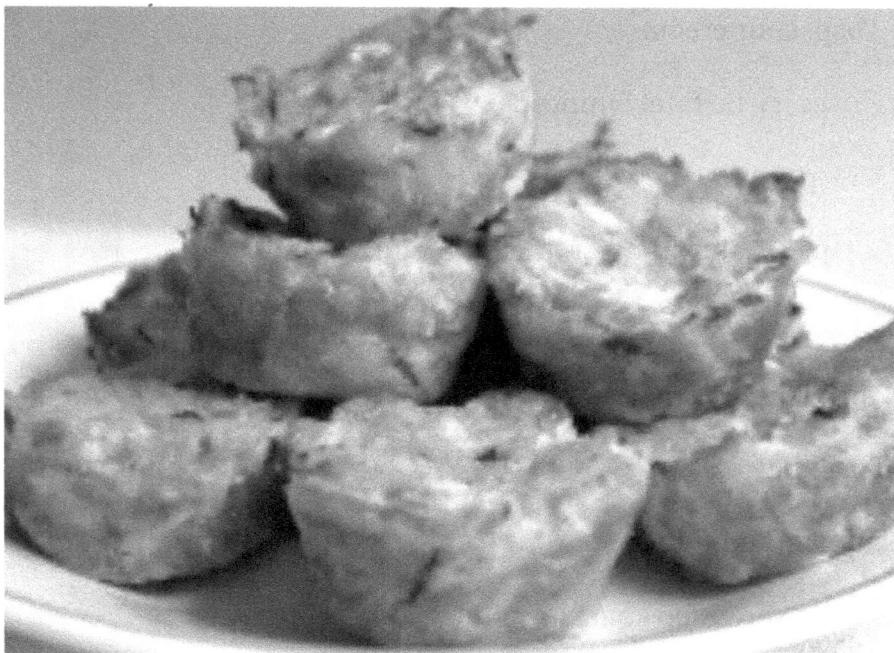

Servings: 28 | **Time:** 30 mins | **Difficulty**: Easy

Nutrients per serving: Calories: 76 kcal | Fat: 6g | Carbohydrates: 2g | Protein: 3g | Fiber: 1g

Ingredients

4 Tbsp. butter melted

3 Tbsp. coconut flour

3 eggs

2 Tbsp. sour cream

2 cloves garlic finely minced

2 ½ tsp. baking powder

1/2 tsp. Monkfruit or Erythritol Blend Sweetener

1 tsp. salt

1 Tbsp. chopped parsley

1 Tbsp. butter

1 cup almond flour

1 ½ cup shredded squash

½ tsp. Pepper

½ cup Colby or Medium Cheddar cheese

¼ tsp. Fiesta Brand-Zesty Italian Delight/Italian Seasoning

¼ cup shredded Parmesan

¼ cup diced onion

Method

1.   Spray and set aside a mini muffin tin or fill a mini muffin tin with liners. Spray well and put aside if you are using the silicone mini muffin tray.

2.   Melt one tbsp of butter in a shallow pan. Garnish with cabbage, rubbed squash, ginger, and 1/2 tsp. Add salt and sauté for 5-7 minutes, just until the onion is shiny. Put aside to cool. There should not be any liquid in the container.

3.   Mix the flour and the next 6 ingredients in a large bowl and mix well to combine. Mix the eggs one at a time. Apply a mixture of melted butter, squash, and sour cream and mix well. Stir the cheese in.

4.   Drop the entire tbsp or put the dough in a ready mini muffin pan using a cookie scoop.

5.   For 20 minutes, bake at 350 F or until the tops are only golden brown. Cool for 5 minutes in a pan, then remove from the pan and cool thoroughly on a rack. They can be eaten warm and also store at room temperature.

38 Roasted Cauliflower Keto Hummus with Red Peppers

Servings: 10 | **Time**: 45 mins | **Difficulty**: Easy

Nutrients per serving: Calories: 137 kcal | Fat: 12g | Carbohydrates: 5g | Protein: 3g | Fiber: 2g

Ingredients

For the Roasted Cauliflower:

3-4 Tbsp. olive (or avocado oil)

1 large head cauliflower (cut into florets)

½ tsp. Garlic powder

½ tsp. cumin

1 tsp. salt

To Finish the Hummus:

2-5 Tbsp. water

2 Tbsp. olive or avocado oil

2 Tbsp. fresh lemon juice

1-2 cloves garlic

1/2 tsp. Cumin

¾ tsp. Salt

¼ tsp. Pepper

¼ cup roasted red pepper

¼ cup + 2 Tbsp. tahini

Method

1.   Preheat the oven to 400°C. Toss the cauliflower florets with olive oil, garlic powder, salt, and cumin in a large cup. Load it onto a sheet pan lined with parchment. Be sure to hit the pan with all the florets for full caramelization. For 30-35 minutes, roast the cauliflower or until the florets become brown and very tender. 5-10 minutes to cool.

2.   Mix the roasted cauliflower, tahini, lemon juice, and the next 6 ingredients in a food processor or the high-speed blender. Puré the mixture until it is smooth. Add a tbsp of water at a time if the hummus is too dense to achieve the target consistency. Serve with keto crackers or vegetables.

39 Keto Spinach Balls

Servings: 16 | **Time:** 30 mins | **Difficulty:** Easy

Nutrients per serving: Calories: 96 kcal | Fat: 8g | Carbohydrates: 1g | Protein: 5g | Fiber: 1g

Ingredients

1/3 cup red onion finely minced

1/3 cup parmesan cheese (finely shredded)

1 Tbsp. butter

3 cloves garlic (finely minced)

1 cup pork rind crumbs

1 tsp. kosher salt

¼ tsp. poultry seasoning

10 oz. frozen spinach (squeezed dried & thawed)

½ cup fontina cheese (finely shredded)

¼ tsp. Black pepper

1 Tbsp. heavy cream

5 Tbsp. butter salted melted

3 eggs

Method

1. Preheat the oven to 350°F. Line up and set aside a large sheet pan.

2. Melt the butter in a small skillet on medium heat. Include the onion then sauté until soft and translucent for 5-7 minutes or when solid. Add garlic and simmer for an additional minute. Remove from the sun and place to cool aside.

3. Mix the dried spinach, cooled onion, pork rind crumbs, garlic, and the next eight ingredients in a medium mixing dish. Mix well and let the mixture sit for 5-10 minutes in the fridge.

4. Divide the mixture into 16 portions using a small scoop, and use your hands to shape each part into a ball. Place balls about an inch apart on the lined cookie sheet and bake for about 15-20 minutes or until they are golden. Take from a sheet pan and put to cool on paper towels. Serve at room temperature or hotter.

40 Cajun Pork Rinds

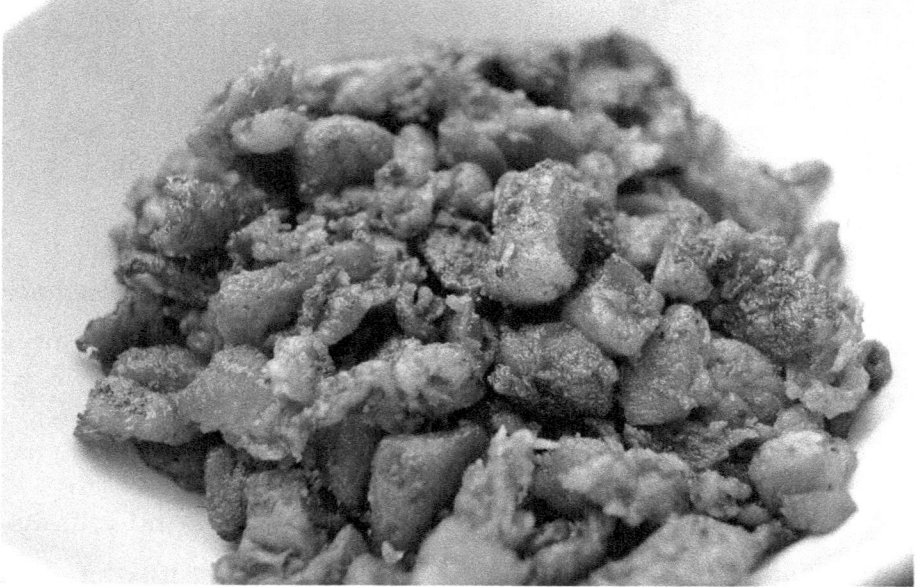

Servings: 14 | **Time**: 1 hr 13 mins | **Difficulty**: Easy

Nutrients per serving: Calories: 51 kcal | Fat: 5g | Carbohydrates: 1g | Protein: 1g | Fiber: 1g

Ingredients

6 Tbsp. melted butter

2 Tbsp. Worcestershire Sauce gluten-free

2 3.25 oz bags of plain pork rinds

1/8 tsp. cayenne pepper

1/2 tsp. paprika

1/2 tsp. onion powder

1/2 tsp. garlic powder

1 1/4 tsp. Fiesta Brand-Cajun All Seasoning

Method

1.   Preheat to 250 F in the oven. Line up and set aside a large sheet pan lined with parchment.

2.   Through a large dish, pour the pork rinds. In a small cup, mix the next 7 ingredients and blend well to mix. Drizzle over the pork rinds with half the butter mixture and toss to cover. Repeat with the mixture of butter that remains. Cover the coasted pork rinds over the pan of prepared sheets and bake for 80 minutes at 250 F, stirring after every 20 minutes.

3.   Take the pork rinds from the oven and pass them to paper towels to make cool. When cold, place at room temperature in an air-tight bag.

Beverages

41   Keto Frozen Blackberry Lemonade

Servings: 2 | **Time**: 5 mins | **Difficulty:** Easy

Nutrients per serving: Calories: 155 kcal | Fat: 15g | Carbohydrates: 6g | Protein: 2g | Fiber: 2g

Ingredients

1 Cup Ice

1/4 Cup Blackberries, Fresh

4 Tbsps. Lemon Juice

1/2 Cup Almond Milk

1/3 Cup Coconut Cream

1 Tbsp. Stevia/Erythritol Blend

1/8 Tsp. Sea Salt

Method

1.   Combine all the ingredients in a blender and mix until a smooth consistency is attained.

2.   Decant into the serving glasses and enjoy.

42   Triple Berry Cheesecake Smoothie

Servings: 1 | **Time**: 5 mins | **Difficulty:** Easy

Nutrients per serving: Calories: 158 kcal | Fat: 11g | Carbohydrates: 12g | Protein: 3g | Fiber: 6g

Ingredients

2 Tbsps. Avocado

1/2 Cup Mixed Berries, Frozen

1 Tsp. Vanilla

2 Tbsps. Cream Cheese

1/8 Tsp. Sea Salt

1/2 Cup Almond Milk, Unsweetened

7-10 Drops Monkfruit Extract

Method

1.   Combine all the ingredients in a blender and mix until a smooth consistency is attained.

2.   Decant into the serving glass and enjoy.

43   Maple Almond Green Smoothie

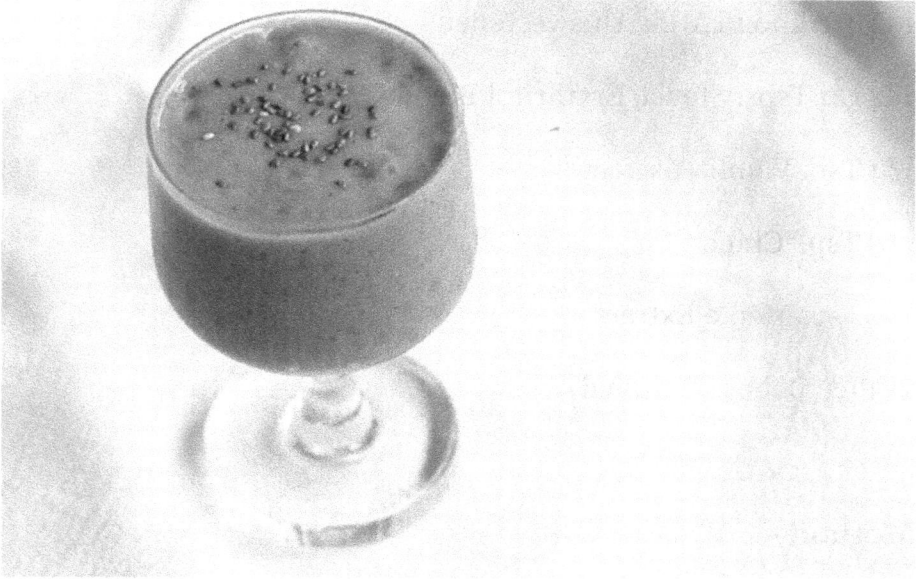

Servings: 1 | **Time:** 5 mins | **Difficulty:** Easy

Nutrients per serving: Calories: 210 kcal | Fat: 16.8g | Carbohydrates: 10.4g | Protein: 8.1g | Fiber: 6.3g

Ingredients

1 Cup Baby Spinach

1 Tbsp. Avocado

1 Tbsp. Golden Flax Meal

1 Tbsp. Almond Butter

1 Cup Almond Milk, Unsweetened

1 & 1/4 Tsps. Stevia/Erythritol Blend

1/4 Tsp. Vanilla Extract

1/8 Tsp. Cinnamon

1/4 Tsp. Maple Extract

2-3 Ice Cubes (Optional)

Method

1.   Combine all the ingredients in a blender and mix until a smooth consistency is attained.

2.   Decant into the serving glass and enjoy.

44 Dairy Free Chocolate Pecan Keto Shake

Servings: 1 | **Time:** 10 mins | **Difficulty**: Easy

Nutrients per serving: Calories: 247 kcal | Fat: 20g | Carbohydrates: 12g | Protein: 5g | Fiber: 8g

Ingredients

5 Raw Pecans, Halved

2 Tbsps. Cocoa Powder, Unsweetened

1/8 Tsp. Pink Himalayan Salt

1 & 1/3 Cups Almond Milk, Unsweetened

2 & 1/2 Tsps. Stevia/Erythritol Blend

2 Tbsps. Avocado

3-4 Ice Cubes

Method

1.   Combine all the ingredients in a blender and mix until a smooth consistency is attained.

2.   Decant into the serving glass and enjoy.

45 Strawberry Colada Milkshake

Servings: 1 | **Time**: 3 mins | **Difficulty**: Easy

Nutrients per serving: Calories: 660 kcal | Fat: 60g | Carbohydrates: 7g | Protein: 13g | Fiber: 7g

Ingredients

1/2 Tbsp. Chia Seeds

3-4 Strawberries, Frozen

1/3 Cup Coconut Milk

1/3 Cup Almond Milk, Unsweetened

1 Tsp. Stevia/Erythritol Blend

4-5 Ice Cubes

1/8 Tsp. Pink Salt

1/4 Tsp. Coconut Extract

1/4 Tsp. Vanilla Extract

1/2 Tbsp. Coconut Oil (Optional)

1 Tbsp. Strawberries, Freeze-Dried (Optional)

Method

1.   Combine all the ingredients in a blender and mix until a smooth consistency is attained.

2.   Decant into the serving glass and enjoy.

46 Keto Frozen Hot Chocolate

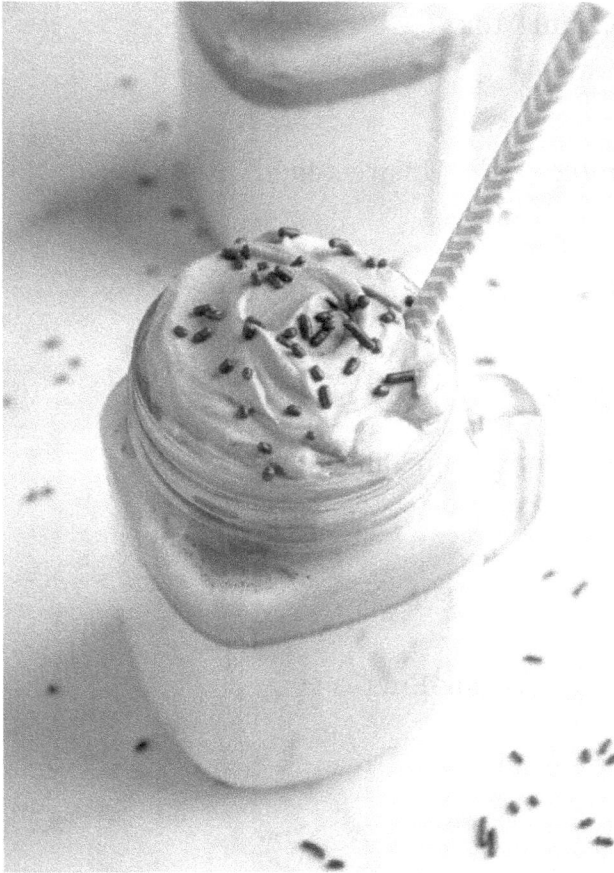

Servings: 1 | **Time:** 5 mins | **Difficulty**: Easy

Nutrients per serving: Calories: 660 kcal | Fat: 60g | Carbohydrates: 7g | Protein: 13g | Fiber: 7g

Ingredients

1 Tbsp. Avocado

1/4 Cup Coconut Milk

1 Tbsp. Cocoa

1/2 Cup Almond Milk, Unsweetened

1/2 Cup Ice Cubes

1 & 1/4 Tsps. Stevia/Erythritol Blend

1/2 Tsp. Vanilla

1/8 Tsp. Pink Himalayan Salt

For Garnish:

Chocolate Chips, Sugar-Free

Whipped Coconut Cream

Method

1.   Combine all the ingredients in a blender except ice cubes. Blend until a smooth consistency is attained.

2.   Decant into the serving glass, add the ice, and put the whipped cream and chocolate chips on top if you want.

47 Dairy-Free Keto Iced Latte

Servings: 1 | **Time:** 5 mins | **Difficulty:** Easy

Nutrients per serving: Calories: 660 kcal | Fat: 60g | Carbohydrates: 7g | Protein: 13g | Fiber: 7g

Ingredients

1/4 Cup Brewed Coffee, Strong

1 & 1/2 Cups Almond Milk, Unsweetened

1 Tbsp. MCT Oil

Method

1.   Brew your coffee according to your preference.

2.   Combine all the ingredients in a blender and mix until a smooth consistency is attained.

3.   Decant into the serving cup and enjoy.

48 Sugar-Free Hibiscus Lemonade

Servings: 4 | **Time:** 10 mins | **Difficulty**: Easy

Nutrients per serving: Calories: 660 kcal | Fat: 60g | Carbohydrates: 7g | Protein: 13g | Fiber: 7g

Ingredients

1 & 1/2 Cups Sparkling Mineral Water

2 Tbsps. Lemon Juice, Fresh

1 Tbsp. Stevia/Erythritol Blend

2 Cups Brewed Hibiscus

Tea Ice, To Taste

Method

1.   Put all the ingredients in a pitcher except water and ice. Mix everything well until dissolved.

2.   Add the water and ice and stir.

3.   Decant into the serving glasses and enjoy.

49   Low Carb 7Up

Servings: 2 | **Time**: 2 mins | **Difficulty:** Easy

Nutrients per serving: Calories: 2 kcal | Fat: 0g | Carbohydrates: 1g | Protein: 0g | Fiber: 0g

Ingredients

1 & 1/2 Cups Ice

1/4 Tsp. Liquid Stevia

1/2 Tbsp. Lime Juice

2/3 Cup Seltzer Water

Method

1.   Fill serving glass with ice and put all the other ingredients in it.

2.   Stir well and enjoy.

50 Low Carb German Chocolate Fat Bomb Hot Chocolate

Servings: 1 | **Time**: 12 mins | **Difficulty**: Easy

Nutrients per serving: Calories: 358 kcal | Fat: 39g | Carbohydrates: 2g | Protein: 2g

Ingredients

2 Tbsps. Cocoa Butter

1/4 Cup Coconut Milk

1 Cup Chocolate Almond Milk,

Unsweetened Stevia, To Taste

Method

1.   In a saucepan, combine all the ingredients and heat over medium-low flame until the cocoa butter melts.

2.   Remove from the heat and mix with an immersion blender till t becomes frothy.

3.   Decant into your favorite mug and enjoy.